Made in United States
Orlando, FL
14 April 2025

60496490R00068